M000192128

The World Is a Small Place

And the smaller it gets, the more important it is that we understand each other.

There's a reason *Cultural Sensitivity* is entering into its third edition and has been expanded to cover religion: The topic of sensitivity in patient-centered care is timeless. It's undeniable that understanding a patient's cultural practices and spiritual beliefs influences not only the delivery of health care in our global society, but also the individual's outcome and satisfaction.

As health care providers in the Western world, we probably understand that every ethnicity on the globe can be found in our major cities—Amsterdam, Berlin, Brussels, Chicago, London, Los Angeles, Madrid, New York, and Paris, to name a few. But what about everywhere else? And does it matter? The answer is an unqualified "absolutely."

Garden City, Kansas, is a community of about 26,000 folks in the southwest part of the state. This small Midwestern town has a population that speaks 21 different languages, not counting English. Jennifer Ng, associate professor of educational leadership and policy studies, and Don Stull, professor emeritus, at the University of Kansas studied this small town and noted, "The very existence of a place like this defies our expectations of what a rural community is." In commenting about the community's schools, Ng said it's "a fascinating place to explore how these changes have mattered as they're one of the few locations where the entire community comes together. They [the schools] are a place of opportunity for the community's children."*

These diverse peoples, regardless of living outside their place of origin, carry with them cultures, customs, and religious beliefs that affect their interpretation of their world, experiences, and relationships—and what they expect when seeking health and wellness.

When it comes to health care, the Western world has great technology and dedicated, intelligent health care staff, but these advantages are lost if patients can't understand the "why" and "what" of their care.

If a patient, because of a cultural or spiritual "disconnect," can't appreciate what is being prescribed or why it's necessary, or if the information is delivered in a way that inadvertently frightens, offends, or confuses the patient, how can we fulfill our mission as health care providers?

Sensitivity is a necessary skill set for health care providers to avoid such disconnects, but even the most dedicated individual can never completely master the skill. **Awareness**—that is, knowledge—is the first step to successful navigation of our world. Once we are aware, we become **accountable** to consciously use or not use what we've learned to improve health care safety, quality, and outcomes for our patients.

The power of awareness and accountability is not limited to application of linear logic to diagnoses and treatments. Somewhat paradoxically, softer aspects of the human condition, such as ethnicity and spirituality, can play a surprisingly big role in a patient's health and well-being—or illness. This then requires health care providers to purposefully educate themselves about these domains so that they can navigate the multicultural environment of their patient population with sensitivity for at least two critically important reasons: (1) It will naturally improve the patient–provider relationship, increasing the likelihood of a good health care outcome; and (2) It is respectful of each patient's specific needs. In brief, paying attention to our patients' ethnicity and spirituality and tailoring our healing approach to needs unveiled by a greater, more holistic understanding are simply good medicine.

*University of Kansas. Garden City Offers Lessons on Education Diverse Populations, Study Says. Nov 15, 2016. Accessed May 14, 2018. https://news.ku.edu/2016/10/31/garden-city-offers-lessons-communities -nationwide-educating-diverse-populations-study.

- Analysis of adverse event data for limited English proficient and English-speaking patients at Joint Commission–accredited hospitals
- Accreditation requirements supporting health equity issues, including communication, culture, religion, and nondiscrimination
- *Advancing Effective Communication, Cultural Competence, and Patient- and Family-Centered Care: A Roadmap for Hospitals*, a monograph with implementation recommendations and examples of practices promoting communication and patient engagement
- *Advancing Effective Communication, Cultural Competence, and Patient- and Family-Centered Care for the Lesbian, Gay, Bisexual, and Transgender (LGBT) Community: A Field Guide*, a publication urging hospitals to create a more welcoming, safe, and inclusive environment for LGBT patients and their families

The resources listed here can be found on the Health Equity portal at the Joint Commission's website at https://www.jointcommission.org/topics/health_equity.aspx. We hope that you find these Joint Commission and JCR resources valuable to you in your efforts to provide the best quality of care to your diverse patient populations.

Christina L. Cordero, PhD, MPH

Project Director
Department of Standards and Survey Methods
Division of Healthcare Quality Evaluation
The Joint Commission

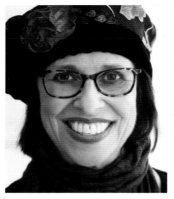

Geri-Ann Galanti, PhD, is a leading expert in the field of cultural diversity, with more than 30 years of experience. She received her doctorate in anthropology from UCLA with an emphasis in medical anthropology. Galanti has been on the faculty of the School of Nursing at Cal State University, Dominguez Hills, and the Anthropology Department at CSU Los Angeles, and is currently teaching in the Doctoring Program at UCLA's David Geffen School of Medicine, where she received an Outstanding Teacher Award. She has written numerous articles, as well as the highly acclaimed book, *Caring for Patients from Different Cultures*, now in its fifth edition.

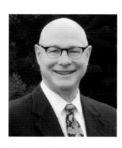

Michael Woods, MD, is a board-certified surgeon and innovative health care leader with a master's degree in medical management and more than 25 years of experience and knowledge in cutting-edge quality measures. Woods has spent more than 15 years focusing on clinical and health information technology (HIT) safety as well as business development, and he has extensive practical knowledge of diverse operational concerns that impact frontline caregivers. The author/contributor of five books, including *Healing Words: The Power of Apology in Medicine* and the first edition of JCR's best-seller, *Cultural Sensitivity*, Woods earned his undergraduate degree in cellular biology, his medical degree, and his surgical training at the University of Kansas. He earned his master's degree at the University of Southern California.

treatments. Most people will try home remedies before coming to a physician; however, few will share such information due to fear of ridicule or chastisement. Because the occasional traditional remedy may be dangerous or could lead to a drug interaction with prescribed medications, it is important that health care providers ask about them. However, it is essential to ask the question in a non-judgmental way, or patients will likely not share such information. Ask in a tone that implies that *of course, everyone tries home remedies before coming in to the doctor*.

4. Concerns: What are your *concerns* regarding the condition and/or recommended treatment? (Perhaps pose questions such as the following: How serious do you think this is? What potential complications do you fear? How does it interfere with your life or your ability to function? Do you know anyone else who has tried the treatment I've recommended? What was their experience with it?)

You want to understand patients' perceptions of the course of the illness and their fears so you can address their concerns and correct any misconceptions. You also want to know what aspects of the condition pose a problem for patients, which may help you uncover something very different from what you might have expected. It is also important to know patients' concerns about any treatment you may prescribe. This can help avoid problems of nonadherence, because some patients may have misplaced concerns based on the experiences of friends and relatives.

ORGANIZATION OF THIS EDITION

This third, expanded edition is separated into two sections; each section starts with a tab labeled *Cultures* and *Religions*, respectively. The goal is to help you quickly and easily access the information you need when you need it.

Anglo-American

Caution: These are broad generalizations and should not be used to stereotype any individuals.

Values, Worldview, and Communication

▸ **Independence is valued,** so patients are likely to be receptive to self-care.
▸ **Both direct eye contact and emotional control are expected.** However, try to avoid excessive direct eye contact with members of the opposite sex to avoid any hint of sexual impropriety.
▸ **Privacy is important,** yet the patient may want/expect nurses to provide psychosocial care.

Time Orientation

▸ **People of lower socioeconomic status tend to be present oriented,** while middle- and upper-class individuals tend to be future oriented.

Pain

▸ **Patients tend to be stoic,** although most will want pain medication. The need for and use of pain medication should be based on the practitioner's discretion when the condition warrants it and after discussing it with the patient.

Family/Gender Issues

▸ **Generally, family size is small, and *immediate family* typically refers to spouse, siblings, parents, and children.** Families are often spread out, and the patient may have fewer visitors than those of other ethnic groups.
▸ **Among LGBTQ patients,** friends may take on a role that is traditionally that of the family in heterosexual Anglo-American culture.
▸ **Husbands and wives usually have equal authority,** with either parent making decisions for the child.

Pregnancy and Birth

▸ **Prenatal care is generally sought.**
▸ **The husband or domestic partner, regardless of gender, is usually the preferred labor partner.**
▸ **Hospital births are generally preferred,** even if an alternative birthing center is used. This may be related to a cultural desire to control events.
▸ **There are no postpartum rituals other than those associated with specific religions.**
▸ **Breast feeding may be practiced for three to six months.**

Anglo-American

Pediatric

▶ **Some upper-middle-class parents believe there is a link between childhood vaccinations and autism** and refuse to get their children vaccinated. Rather than telling them studies have shown there's no connection between vaccines and autism, it may be more helpful to focus on the diseases the vaccines prevent and how these diseases can harm their children. Spacing out the timing of giving vaccines may make them more acceptable to parents.

End of Life

▶ **Patients will generally want to know their diagnosis and prognosis.**

▶ **Although many want "everything done," hospice is usually an acceptable alternative.** Often, however, hospice is not seriously pursued until the last few days before death. Some people mistakenly believe that they will receive no medical care if they are on hospice. Be sure to discuss their concerns when you first introduce the concept of hospice.

▶ **Stoicism is valued when someone dies.** A lack of emotional expression does not necessarily reflect a lack of feeling.

▶ **Organ donations and autopsies are acceptable,** as are cremation or burial unless forbidden by the patient's religion.

Health Beliefs and Practices

▶ **A patient may prefer to be left alone when ill.**

▶ **Patients generally prefer an aggressive approach to treating illness.**

▶ **Biomedicine is preferred, although many may also use complementary and alternative medicine.** Be sure to inquire—in a nonjudgmental way—about the use of herbal medications.

▶ **Germs are thought to cause disease, and patients expect treatment to destroy germs.** Antibiotics are often requested, even for treating viral illnesses. Be sure to explain the difference between treating viral and bacterial conditions. Explain why antibiotics must be finished, even after symptoms subside.

▶ **Middle-class patients commonly use the Internet to obtain information** and may want to dictate specific treatment based on what they learn from that source. Suggest reputable Internet sources they can use if they want more information.

Asian

Caution: These are broad generalizations and should not be used to stereotype any individuals. They are most applicable to the least acculturated members. Individuals from China, Japan, Korea, and the Philippines are included in this group.

Values, Worldview, and Communication

▸ **Harmony and avoidance of conflict are highly valued.** For this reason, patients may agree to things on which they have no intention of following through. Similarly, agreement may also be offered out of respect. Make sure the reasons for any directives or recommendations are explained and stressed. Avoid asking questions requiring a "yes" or "no" response. Find a way to have the patient demonstrate an understanding of what you expect.

▸ **Filial piety (respect for and duty to one's parents) is an important value.** This may make end-of-life conversations with adult children more complicated, as children may not want to be seen as "giving up" on their parents.

▸ **As a sign of respect, patients might avoid direct eye contact.** Do not assign other meanings to this.

▸ **Avoid hand gestures in case they are offensive.** For example, beckoning with the index finger may be insulting to Filipinos and Koreans, because it is a gesture commonly used to call dogs.

▸ **Giggling at "inappropriate" times usually indicates nervousness or discomfort.** Do not assume a lack of seriousness.

▸ **Make offers several times,** as patients may refuse at first to be polite.

▸ **Pronouns do not exist in most Asian languages,** so some patients might confuse *he* and *she*.

Time Orientation

▸ **Time orientation varies among Asian cultures.** Traditional Chinese patients may be past oriented, placing a heavy value on tradition. Filipinos may be both past and present oriented and may not always adhere to *clock time*. Japanese may be both past and future oriented, and generally on time. Many Koreans are future oriented and adhere to clock time for appointments but not social events.

Asian

Pain

▶ **Stoicism is highly valued.** Pain may be expressed only by a clenched jaw. The need for and use of pain medication should be based on the practitioner's discretion when the condition warrants it and after discussing it with the patient.

▶ **Filipinos may be particularly concerned about addiction to pain medication.** If they do not ask for pain medications or refuse them when offered, ask them about their concerns so you can clarify any misunderstandings.

Family/Gender Issues

▶ **Most Asian cultures tend to be hierarchical,** with the elderly afforded more respect than younger people, and males more than females. Accept that wives may defer to husbands in decision making and that sons may be valued more than daughters.

▶ **Allow family members to spend as much time as possible with the patient,** as many consider it their familial duty. Involve the family in decision making when it comes to the patient's care.

▶ **Traditionally, wives are expected to care for their husbands, which may interfere with self-care.** If some aspects of self-care are medically necessary, give the wife another task—such as rubbing lotion on her husband's hands or feet—as a way for her to help her spouse.

Pregnancy and Birth

▶ **Traditionally, the birth partner was the mother-in-law or another female relative and may still be true** for recent immigrants.

▶ **Because pregnancy is thought to be a yang or "hot" condition in traditional Chinese medicine, birth is believed to deplete the body of heat.** Restoration of warmth is important. With this in mind, offer new mothers liquids other than ice water, which may be deemed too yin or "cold." The new mother may want traditional soups or foods. Offer them, if possible, or allow family members to bring them in. Also, respect postpartum prescriptions for rest.

▶ **Traditionally, bathing is avoided for a month after giving birth.** If a patient is reluctant to shower, offer a sponge bath.

Asian

▸ **Parents may avoid naming the baby for up to 30 days.** Traditionally, a child is given an unattractive nickname before then to avoid attracting the attention of spirits who might want to steal the child.

Pediatric

▸ **A great deal of pressure is often put on children to succeed in school.**

▸ **"Mongolian spots" are common in Asian babies and should not be misinterpreted as bruises.** This congenital birthmark usually fades as the infant grows into childhood.

End of Life

▸ **When patients are diagnosed as terminal, family members may wish to shield them from that fact.** Upon admission (or before the need arises, if possible), ask patients how much information they want regarding their condition, or to whom the information should be provided. If the patient requests that all information be given to a family member, be sure to investigate the legal implications of doing so according to the HIPAA (Health Insurance Portability and Accountability Act of 1996) law, which provides for patient privacy of medical information. Be aware that in most parts of Asia, diagnoses are usually given to the family, who decide whether or not to tell the patient.

▸ **Patients and their families may not want to discuss end-of-life issues in advance.** If it is important to have such conversations, approach them respectfully, saying something such as, "I know that some families don't like to discuss these issues in advance. Is this something that you feel comfortable discussing with me?"

▸ **Cancer is both highly feared and stigmatized.** If patients have indicated that they do not want to know their diagnosis, subsequent discussions should involve terms such as *growth* or *lesion* rather than *cancer* or *tumor*, and *medication* rather than *chemotherapy*.

▸ **Due to the high level of respect for parents and the elderly, some adult children may be reluctant to withdraw life support** for fear of giving the appearance of not honoring their parents.

Asian

Health Beliefs and Practices

▶ **In China and Korea, coining and cupping therapies are traditional medical practices** and not forms of abuse, despite the marks these practices may leave on a patient's body. Ask about any suspicious-looking marks before making any assumptions.

▶ **Fevers are often treated by covering the patient in warm blankets and offering warm liquids.** If it is medically necessary to do the opposite, try to compromise (for example, ice blanket with warm liquids) and explain the reason for your actions without insulting their beliefs.

▶ **Avoid giving ice water without asking if the patient prefers it to water at room temperature.** Patients may prefer hot liquids, such as tea. Offer several options.

▶ **The use of herbs is common.** If patients have used only traditional Chinese herbs, they may not know how to take Western medications, because the herbs are usually boiled in water and then drunk. In that situation, be sure to explain how to use the medications and provide written directions as necessary.

▶ **Avoid the number 4.** Because the character for the number 4 is pronounced the same as the character for the word *death* in several Asian languages, avoid putting these patients in rooms or operating rooms identified with that number if possible.

▶ **Mental illness can be highly stigmatizing in Asian countries.** Patients with emotional problems are likely to present with physical complaints. They may be reluctant to discuss emotional problems with anyone outside the family, including health care professionals. Although counterintuitive, assigning providers of the same ethnic background may be less effective due to (unwarranted) concern that the providers will talk about them within the community. Framing emotional problems in terms of physical complaints may be helpful. For example, you might say, "Stomachaches can be caused by stress. Tell me about what's going on in your life."

Black American

Note: At the time of printing, "Black American" and "African American" are both currently in use. We've chosen to use Black American for this edition to distinguish American-born blacks from those who were born in African countries. Be aware, however, that your American-born patient may prefer the term African American to Black American.

Values, Worldview, and Communication

▸ **Black American patients, particularly older ones, may not trust hospitals,** due to a long history of racism and discrimination. Also, they may be aware of current studies documenting racial disparities in health care. Sometimes it can help to ask directly about their concerns.

▸ **Black Americans may be very sensitive to discrimination, even when it is not intended.** For example, do not use the term *gal* to refer to a woman. It has the same connotations as *boy* for a Black American male. Address the patient as Mr., Mrs., or Ms., or by professional title and last name. As with all patients, apologize and explain if a patient is kept waiting, or it may be interpreted as a sign of disrespect or discrimination.

▸ **Religion is important to many Black Americans.** Clergy should be allowed to participate when appropriate. Privacy and quiet time for prayer are important. Health care practitioners may offer to pray with a patient if all parties are comfortable. It is customary for clergy and acquaintances from the patient's place of worship to visit the sick on Sundays, often directly from church. Don't assume all Black Americans practice the same religion. For more on a specific religion, *see* the section on religions at the end of this guide.

Time Orientation

▸ **Those of lower socioeconomic status may have a present time orientation, which may impede preventive medicine and follow-up care.** Explain the need for preventive medication (such as for hypertension) or to finish antibiotics even when symptoms disappear. Some may delay seeing a physician until symptoms are severe.

Pain

▸ **Expressions of pain vary widely.** It is equally acceptable to be expressive or stoic.

Black American

Family/Gender Issues

▶ **Family structure may be nuclear, extended, or matriarchal.** Close friends or church members may be considered kin and even referred as "sister" or "brother." Households headed by women are common. In such cases, a grandmother or aunt may be the patient's spokesperson. Often, the father or eldest male may take this role.

▶ **Generally, women are considered equal to men.** Many women achieve higher socioeconomic status and educational levels than men.

Pregnancy and Birth

▶ **Prenatal care is common.**

▶ **Traditionally, only females attended birth, but this now varies.** Today, a male partner often assists the delivery.

End of Life

▶ **The incidence and death rates for some types of cancer, including prostate and cervical, are particularly high among Black Americans.** This may be due in part to the lack of trust in the health care system that leads to delays in screening.

▶ **Patients may be reluctant to sign a DNR (do not resuscitate) order for fear that physicians will withhold beneficial treatment.** If they are reluctant, you might say, "Sometimes patients are afraid that if they sign a DNR, doctors will withhold treatment that could help them. Is this something you're concerned about?"

▶ **There may be reluctance to remove life support due to a belief in miracles.** The thought may be that God may create a miracle and save the patient. Another source of reluctance may be distrust for the medical community. If they are reluctant, the best approach may be to discuss it with them. For example, you might say, "Sometimes patients don't want to remove life support because they believe God may create a miracle. Sometimes it's because they don't trust us. Is this something you're concerned about? Do you have other concerns about removing life support?"

▶ **Some consider it taboo to donate organs or blood except to a family member, for fear it will hasten one's own death.** If patients are reluctant, the best approach may be to discuss it with them. You might say, "Sometimes patients don't want to donate organs or

Black American

blood because they fear it will cause them to die sooner. Is this something you're concerned about? Do you have other concerns about donating organs (blood)?"

Health Beliefs and Practices

▸ **Some may believe that disease is a punishment for sin.** Be sure to ask patients what they think caused their disease, and if they say it is punishment for sin, it may be helpful to involve clergy or to have the patient pray for God to guide the physicians.

▸ **The Black American culture has a rich tradition of herbal remedies.** Be sure to discuss the use of home or herbal remedies to prevent potential drug interactions. It is important to ask, in a nonjudgmental way, implying that of course everyone tries home remedies before coming in to see the doctor.

Note: Material is drawn from the work of Loudell Snow on African Americans of lower socioeconomic status in the rural South, as well as Waters CM, Locks S. African Americans. In Lipson JG, Dibble SL, editors: Culture & Clinical Care. *San Francisco: UCSF Nursing Press, 2005, 14–26; and National Cancer Institute.* Cancer Health Disparities. *Mar 11, 2008. Accessed May 14, 2018. http://www.cancer.gov/cancer-topics/factsheet/cancer-health-disparities.*

Middle Eastern

▸ **Injections may be preferable to pills** based on the belief that injections are more effective. Offer options when available.

▸ **Damp, cold, and drafts may be thought to lead to illness.** Strong emotions are also suspect. For example, the "evil eye" (usually motivated by envy) may be thought to cause illness or misfortune. Amulets to prevent this may be worn and should not be removed.

▸ **The patient may feel slighted if not given a prescription.**

▸ **Observant Muslims do not eat pork.** Muslims are also expected to abstain from alcohol, which may be in cough medicine. Medications that contain gelatin may also be a problem.

▸ **If a patient or family member offers you food, it may be perceived as rude to refuse it.** After it is offered twice (indicating it was a sincere rather than merely polite offer), it's best to accept it graciously.

Note: Some of this information is based on material from Meleis Al. Arabs. In Lipson JG, Dibble SL, editors: Culture & Clinical Care. San Francisco: UCSF Nursing Press, 2005, 42–57; and Hafizi H. Iranians. In Lipson JG, Dibble SL, editors: Culture & Clinical Care. San Francisco: UCSF Nursing Press, 2005, 264–276.

Middle Eastern

End of Life

- **When offering chemotherapy, offer all options for administration.** Although an implantable pump may seem the most convenient, it may be determined that it has rendered a Muslim "unclean," thus preventing him or her from praying.
- **When a patient is diagnosed as terminal, family may wish to shield him or her from that fact.** Upon admission (or before the need arises), ask patients to identify how much information they want regarding their condition, or to whom the information should be provided.
- **Patients may not want to plan for death** because doing so can be seen as challenging the will of Allah. It may be helpful to say, "I know that some people don't want to make plans for their death because they see it as challenging the will of God. Is this something that concerns you? May we talk about it?"
- **Avoidance of planning for death may interfere with acceptance of hospice care.** Also, they may believe that the family should care for the patient. When discussing hospice, explain that it can be done at home.
- **Muslims may not allow organ donation,** as tradition dictates that the body should be returned to Allah as it was given: whole. Those in favor say that because it can save a life, it falls under the Islamic doctrine that "necessity allows the prohibited." For the same reason, they may not allow an autopsy but will if required by law.

Health Beliefs and Practices

- **Muslims may not take medications, eat, or drink from sunrise to sunset during Ramadan.** This month of fasting, self-sacrifice, and introspection is based on the Islamic calendar and thus occurs at a different time each year. Although they may be exempt during illness or pregnancy, they may have to make up for it later, when friends and family are not observing the practice, making it more difficult for them. Make sure the physician adjusts their medications to any changes in eating patterns.
- **Family members are often expected to take care of patients.** Because of this, include family members in any patient education.

All forms of spirituality (used synonymously with *religion* in this Foreword), lived authentically, exude compassion, inclusiveness, kindness, respect, and service for our fellow human beings. To my way of thinking, these qualities describe the goals—if not the core requirements—of health care delivery. If the reader accepts this as true, then there is no circumstance in which delivery of safe, high-quality care should be denied, limited, or altered due to a patient's—or provider's—religious or spiritual beliefs, any more than care should be denied, limited, or altered due to ethnicity.

How Do We Do This?

As health care providers, we must work within the laws governing our profession (such as HIPAA*), but we cannot hide behind laws or rigid personal beliefs, ignoring the well-accepted moral and ethical imperatives of the healing profession: *Primum non nocere*. "First, do no harm" applies holistically to our patients' well-being—mind, body, culture, and spirit. People go to providers for help, and we need to help them however they show up, even if it means we need to help them find a provider who can deliver care within patients' specific spiritual and cultural needs.

That will result in our patients feeling understood and respected, and they'll be more likely to trust and comply with prescribed therapies and treatments. Safer, higher-quality health care with better outcomes will follow as a natural consequence of doing the right thing.

This third edition, now titled *Cultural and Religious Sensitivity: A Pocket Guide for Health Care Professionals[†]*, has been expanded to include religion and is a wide-open door to the awareness health care providers need to understand their patients' diverse cultural and spiritual perspectives and needs. The only requirement is for health care providers to walk through it, eyes and minds wide open, and be willing to hold themselves accountable for being sensitive to what they learn.

—*Michael S. Woods, MD*

[†]*This expanded edition of the pocket guide is also available as an app from the App Store and Google Play.*

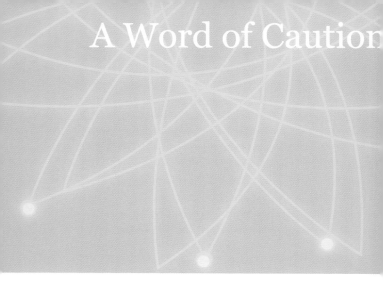

GENERALIZATIONS SHOULD NOT BE MISTAKEN FOR STEREOTYPES.

If I meet Rosa, a Mexican woman, and say to myself, "Rosa is Mexican; she must have a large family," I am stereotyping her. However, if I think, "Mexicans often have large families," and then ask Rosa how many people are in her family, I am making a generalization.

A **stereotype** is an ending point. No attempt is made to learn whether the individual in question fits the statement. Given the tremendous variation within each culture and religion, stereotypes are often incorrect and can have negative results.

A **generalization** is a beginning point. It indicates common trends, but further information is needed to ascertain whether the statement is appropriate to an individual. Generalizations may be inaccurate when applied to specific individuals, but when applied broadly, they can indicate common behaviors and shared beliefs. They can be helpful in suggesting possible avenues to consider and questions to ask.

A FEW FUNDAMENTALS

Let's look at some core causes for cultural "disconnects" between health care providers and patients, beginning with **values**. Simply put: Different cultures and religions promote different values.

Right now, Western culture values such things as money, freedom, independence, privacy, health and fitness, and physical appearance. But another culture—say, the Mbuti of central Africa—might value social support. To punish a wrongdoer, US courts may take the person's money (through a fine of some sort) or the person's freedom (through incarceration). The Mbuti, on the other hand, punish wrongdoers by ignoring them. When a health care system makes decisions based on finances, people from a social-centric culture like the Mbuti may not "get it."

Similarly, in the United States the value of independence is evident in children moving away from home as soon as they are financially able. In other cultures, children might not move out until they are married and often not even then. Health care providers might expect patients to take care of themselves without considering the role of family members in the dynamics of the individual's daily activities of life. For example, nurses encouraging "self-care" might want to consider the home situation to which a patient will be returning, and, when appropriate, distinguish between self-care that is medically necessary and self-care that is merely an imposition of dominant culture values.

Because privacy is also important in Western cultures, the United States enacted HIPAA (Health Insurance Portability and Accountability Act of 1996), which provides for privacy of medical information. This can create problems for people who come from cultures in which the family, rather than the individual, is the primary unit. Family members may pressure health providers to give them information about the patient, and may even ask the provider to withhold information from the patient. Similarly, some cultures value self-control, but some patients come from cultures in which emotional expressiveness is the norm.

Similar illustrations could be made for all the things people value. But the point is that understanding people's values is key to understanding their behavior, because people's behavior generally reflects their values.

TIME ORIENTATION

Time orientation—one's focus regarding time—varies from culture to culture. No individual or culture will look exclusively to the past, present, or future, but most will tend to emphasize one over the others.

Past-oriented cultures are traditional and believe in doing things the way they have always been done. These cultures usually prefer traditional approaches to healing rather than accepting each new procedure or medication that comes out. People with a predominantly present time orientation may be less likely to utilize preventive health measures. They may reason that there is no point in taking a pill for hypertension when they feel fine, particularly if the pill is expensive and causes unpleasant side effects. They may not look ahead in hope of preventing a stroke or heart attack, or they may feel they will deal with it when it happens.

Poverty often forces people into a present time orientation. They are not likely to make plans for the future when they are concerned with surviving today. Time orientation can also refer to degree of adherence to clock time versus adherence to activities. From the perspective of one oriented to the clock, someone who arrives at 3:15 for a 2:30 appointment is late. For someone who does not focus on clock time, both represent midafternoon. To this person, the time to arrive at an afternoon appointment is after the morning activity is completed.

SOCIAL STRUCTURE

The US model of social structure is egalitarian, which in theory means that everyone is equal. Status and power come from an individual's achievements rather than from age, gender, family, or occupation. Other cultures, such as Asian, are hierarchical, where everyone is not considered equal. Status comes from age, gender, and occupation, and these differences are considered important.

RELEVANT ANTHROPOLOGICAL CONCEPTS

One way to discuss the impact of culture on our thinking and behavior is through two anthropological concepts:

1. ETHNOCENTRISM, which is the view that the way of doing things in one's own culture is the right and natural way to do them. Most humans are ethnocentric; that is only natural. But ethnocentrism can impede cross-cultural communication and understanding.

2. CULTURAL RELATIVISM, which is the attitude that other ways of doing things are different but equally valid. This is the attitude we should all strive for, in most cases, as it will lead to better communication and trust.

The practitioners of Western health care tend to believe that their approaches to healing are superior to all others. But the goal of all healing is the same: to help people get well. If different cultures studied each other's techniques with an open mind, the cause of modern medicine would be greatly advanced.

Poor health outcomes are often associated with lack of adherence. Trust is an important key to adherence. One avenue to creating trust is for the health care provider to demonstrate concern for and understanding of the patient's perspective. The best way to achieve that is to ask some important questions, and then listen—really listen—to the answers.

RELIGION AND SPIRITUALITY

Throughout the first half of this guide, and under the headings "End of Life" and "Health Beliefs and Practices," we touch on some religious beliefs of particular cultural groups and how those beliefs may affect patient-centered care. For those who are religious, their religion shapes their values and their worldview as well as their behavior to a great extent. However, people may be spiritual without belonging to an organized religion. In this third and expanded edition, although the focus is on organized religions, it is important to acknowledge that each person's spiritual beliefs are going to be very different.

As you explore this new content, bear in mind that the discussions of religion are meant to be generalizations; not every member of a religious group will necessarily follow any or all of the guidelines advocated by their religion. In addition, in some cultures there may be a predominant religion, but health care professionals encounter people from multiple diverse cultures who may practice the same religion differently based on their individual spirituality. Health care providers may use this information as a starting point from which to ask questions to ascertain their individual patient's beliefs and practices.
DO NOT STEREOTYPE!

Some questions you can ask your patients include the following:[‡]

▸ Do you have any spiritual beliefs that help you cope with stress?
▸ Have your beliefs influenced how you take care of yourself while ill?
▸ Are you part of a spiritual or religious community? (If so), is this community of support to you, and how?
▸ Are there religious issues you would like me to address in your health care?
▸ Are there spiritual practices health care providers can help you keep? For example, special prayer times?
▸ Are there religious articles you would like to use, wear, or keep close?
▸ Are there special rites or blessings for the sick?
▸ Are there any spiritual or religious leaders you would find helpful to bring in?
▸ Are there dietary rules that you follow?

‡Questions adapted from Saguil A, Phelps K. The spiritual assessment. Am Fam Physician. 2012 Sep 15;86(6):546–550. Accessed May 14, 2018. https://www.aafp.org/afp/2012/0915/p546.html; and Diversity Services, Fraser Health Authority. Questions You Can Ask to Understand the Beliefs, Values and Needs of Your Patient/Client/Resident. Accessed May 14, 2018. https://www.fraser-health.ca/media/Understanding-beliefs-culture.pdf.

THE 4 *C'S* OF CULTURALLY SENSITIVE CARE: A MNEMONIC FOR HEALTH CARE PROFESSIONALS[§]

One way to remember what questions to ask is to use the following mnemonic:

1. Call: What do you *call* your problem? (Remember to ask, "What do *you* think is wrong?" This gets at the patient's perception of the problem. You should *not* literally ask, "What do you call your problem?")

The same symptoms may have very different meanings in different cultures and may result in barriers to compliance. For example, among Asia's Hmong people, epilepsy is described as "the spirit catches you, and you fall down."[||] Seeing epilepsy as spirit possession (which has some positive connotations for the possessed) is very different from seeing it as a disruption of the electrical signals in the brain. This might lead to a very different doctor-patient conversation and might help explain why such a patient may be less anxious than the physician to stop the seizures. Understanding the patient's point of view can help the health care provider deal with potential barriers to compliance.

2. Cause: What do you think *caused* your problem? (This gets at the patient's beliefs regarding the source of the problem.)

Not everyone believes that disease is caused by germs. In some cultures, it is thought to be caused by an upset in body balance, a breach of taboo (similar to what is seen in some cultures as diseases due to "sin" and punishment by God), or spirit possession. Treatment must be appropriate to the cause, or people will not perceive themselves as cured. Physicians thus need to find out what the patient believes caused the problem and treat that as well. For example, it may sometimes be appropriate to bring in clergy to pray with the patient if he patient believes God is punishing him or her for some transgression.

3. Cope: How do you *cope* with your condition? (This is to remind the practitioner to ask, "What have you done to try to make it better? Who else have you been to for treatment?")

This will provide the health care provider with important information on the possible use of alternative healers and

§Developed by Stuart Slavin, MD; Geri-Ann Galanti, PhD; and Alice Kuo, MD.

||Fadiman A. The Spirit Catches You and You Fall Down. *New York, NY: Noonday Press. 1997.*

Native American

Caution: These are broad generalizations and should not be used to stereotype any individuals. There are more than 550 different Native American tribes, with much variation among them.

Values, Worldview, and Communication

- **Anecdotes or metaphors may be used by patients to describe their own health.** For example, a story about an ill neighbor may be the patient's way of saying that he or she has the same symptoms.
- **Long pauses often indicate that careful consideration is being given to a question.** Do not rush the patient.
- **Both loudness and a firm handshake are often associated with aggressiveness and should be avoided.**
- **Lack of direct eye contact could be a sign of respect** or possibly a desire to avoid loss or theft of one's soul. Do not misinterpret it as lack of interest or evasiveness.
- **Due to a history of misuse of signed documents, some Native American patients may be unwilling to sign informed consent or advance directives.** In fact, some may be hostile to health care providers due to the history of poor treatment of Native Americans. Be sure to listen to and talk with them about their concerns.
- **The names of deceased relatives may be avoided,** though a relationship term (for example, "brother," "father," "sister") may be used instead.

Time Orientation

- **A present time orientation is common.** Patients are generally oriented to activities rather than to the clock.

Pain

- **These patients generally tend to be stoic,** not expressing pain other than by mentioning, "*I don't feel so good*" or "*Something doesn't feel right.*" The need for and use of pain medication should be based on the practitioner's discretion when the condition warrants it and after discussing it with the patient.

Family/Gender Issues

- **Extended family is important, and any illness concerns the entire family.** Be sure to ask the patient if he or she would like family members included in any discussions.
- **Decision making varies with kinship structure.** Patients generally make their own decisions.

Native American

Pregnancy and Birth

▶ **Prenatal care is uncommon.**
▶ **A female relative may be the birth attendant.** Stoicism is encouraged during labor and delivery.
▶ **Postpartum, the mother and infant may stay inside and rest for 20 days** or until the umbilical cord falls off, depending on custom. Some may want to save the umbilical cord because it may be seen as having spiritual value.

Pediatric

▶ **In some tribes, long, thick hair is the sign of a healthy child; cutting it is taboo and believed to lead to illness or even death. Check with the family before cutting a child's hair.**
▶ **Teen pregnancy rates are high** and may be more culturally acceptable than in other populations.

End of Life

▶ **Some tribes may prefer to avoid discussion of a terminal prognosis or a DNR (do not resuscitate) order** because they believe that negative thoughts hasten death. Others will use the information to make appropriate preparations. If a patient does appear to avoid the subject, you might say, "I know that some people have serious concerns about discussing the end of life. Do you share those concerns? May we talk about them?"
▶ **Some tribes may avoid contact with the dying,** while others may want to be at the bedside 24 hours a day. Visitors may display a jovial attitude so as not to demoralize the patient. Mourning is often done in private, away from the patient.
▶ **After death, wailing and shrieking may occur.**
▶ **Some may want to leave a window open for the soul to leave at death;** others may orient the patient's body to a cardinal direction before death.

Native American

Health Beliefs and Practices

- **Before cutting or shaving hair, check to see if the patient or family wants to keep it.** Realize that in some tribes, cutting hair is associated with mourning.
- **A medicine bag may be worn by the patient.** Do not treat it casually or remove it without discussing it with the patient. If it is absolutely necessary to remove it, allow a family member to do so, keep it as close to the patient as possible, and return it as soon as possible.
- **Food that is blessed (in a traditional religion or Christianity) may be thought to be harmless.** Nutritional guidance should take this into account. Many traditional foods are high in fat.
- **Similarly, tobacco is seen as sacred and has important ceremonial use in some tribes.** This may be a challenge when counseling against smoking. It may be helpful to focus on the sacramental uses of tobacco, in contrast to the habit of smoking.
- **A traditional ritual that may be used for healing is the sweat lodge.** It is akin to an outdoor sauna and involves long rounds of prayer while sweating.
- **Traditional healers may be combined with the use of Western medicine.** Allow traditional healers to perform rituals whenever possible.

Note: Much information is adapted from Kramer J. American Indians. In Lipson JG, Dibble SL, Minarik PA, editors: Culture & Clinical Care: A Pocket Guide. San Francisco: UCSF Nursing Press, 1996, 11–22; and Palacios J, Butterfly R, Strickland CJ. American Indians/Alaskan Natives. In Lipson JG, Dibble SL, editors: Culture & Clinical Care. San Francisco: UCSF Nursing Press, 2005, 27–41.

Russian

Caution: These are broad generalizations and should not be used to stereotype any individuals. They are most applicable to the least acculturated members.

Values, Worldview, and Communication

▸ **To help allay the anxiety of family, provide frequent updates on treatments and progress.** Patients may expect nurses to be friendly, warm, and caring—that is, to "feel" for them.

▸ **Family and friends are expected to visit patients in the hospital;** they may participate in providing care. Family may want to stay overnight.

▸ **They may speak loudly;** this was likely necessary in Russia to get attention in the health care system.

▸ **Make direct eye contact, be firm, and be respectful.** Address patients using their last names preceded by Mr., Mrs., or Ms.

▸ **They tend to be very direct and straightforward** and do not spend time on small talk.

Time Orientation

▸ **These patients are mostly future oriented,** and punctuality is valued. They may arrive early to appointments to be seen first, or late in the day so as to not waste time waiting.

Pain

▸ **These patients generally tend to be very stoic.** They also may fear drug addiction, so the need for and decision to use pain medication should be based on the practitioner's discretion if the condition warrants it and after discussing it with the patient.

Family/Gender Issues

▸ **Patients often have a strong extended family,** with mothers and the elderly often well regarded.

▸ **The sex of the provider is usually not an issue,** but a patient may prefer to have a family member of the same sex present when receiving personal care.

Pregnancy and Birth

▸ **Exercise and lifting heavy objects are often avoided during pregnancy** for fear of harming the unborn baby.

▸ **A female relative is often the preferred labor and delivery partner.**

Russian

End of Life

- **Autopsies and organ donations may be refused** due to what may be considered the sacredness of the body.
- **When patients are diagnosed as terminal, family members may wish to shield them from that fact.** Upon admission (or before the need arises) ask patients how much information they want regarding their condition, or to whom the information should be provided.
- **These patients generally accept hospice care.**

Health Beliefs and Practices

- **Many, particularly the elderly, believe that illness results from cold.** Therefore, keep a patient covered, close windows, keep the room warm, and avoid iced drinks, particularly if the patient has a fever. These patients may also prefer sponge baths to showers.
- **They may not like taking a large number of pills.** Space out medication administration so that as few pills as possible are given at one time.
- **They may prefer nonpharmacologic interventions for nausea,** including lemon slices, ginger ale, mineral water, or weak tea with lemon. Be sure to offer choices.
- **They may practice cupping therapy,** so any resulting marks should not be misinterpreted as abuse or a symptom. Be sure to ask about the marks before making any assumptions.

Note: Information in this profile is based on the work of Peter Anderson, RN, and from Evanikoff del Puerto L, Sigal E. Russians and others from the former Soviet Union.. In Lipson JG, Dibble SL, editors: Culture & Clinical Care. *San Francisco: UCSF Nursing Press, 2005, 415–430.*

South Asian

Caution: These are broad generalizations and should not be used to stereotype any individuals. They are most applicable to the least acculturated members. People from India, Pakistan, Bangladesh, Sri Lanka, and Nepal are included in this group.

Values, Worldview, and Communication

▶ **Hindus and Sikhs may believe illness is the result of karma,** due to actions in a past life. Those who follow Ayurvedic medicine may see it as resulting from an imbalance in bodily humors. (For more on Hinduism and Sikhism, *see* the appropriate tabs in the Religions section later in this guide.)

▶ **Patients may not express feelings openly,** so observe facial expressions closely.

▶ **Direct eye contact may be considered rude or disrespectful,** particularly among the elderly, so do not misinterpret it negatively.

▶ **Silence often indicates acceptance or approval.** With some South Asians, a side-to-side head bob may indicate agreement or uncertainty. An up-and-down nod may indicate disagreement, while acknowledging what the speaker is saying.

▶ **Some patients may not want to sign consents,** as they may consider health care professionals to be the authorities and thus may prefer to have the providers make the decisions. Ask them about their concerns and explain your reasoning for any recommendations.

Time Orientation

▶ **This group is generally future oriented.** Some, including some Pakistanis, may not be oriented to clock time.

Pain

▶ **These patients generally tend to be stoic,** except during childbirth. Pain management should be left to the practitioner's discretion.

▶ **There is a great concern regarding drug addiction,** and thus there may be a reluctance to take pain medication. Pain management should be left to the practitioner's discretion. When pain medication is necessary, practitioners should explain why and address concerns and misunderstandings. Muslims may not want narcotics for anything other than severe pain.

▶ **Some Pakistani Muslims may prefer injections to pills.**

South Asian

Family/Gender Issues

▸ **Women are often modest** and may prefer a gown that provides better coverage. Many may prefer female caregivers as well.

▸ **Male health care providers should not shake hands with a female** unless she offers her hand first.

▸ **Close female family members may insist on remaining with the patient.** Family members may take over the activities of daily living for the patient, such as feeding, grooming, and so on. Because of this, do not insist that the patient practice self-care unless medically necessary.

▸ **The father or eldest son usually has decision-making power,** but generally family members are consulted before decisions are made. Husbands may answer questions addressed to their wives. This does not necessarily indicate an abusive situation.

Pregnancy and Birth

▸ **Pregnant Hindu women are often encouraged to eat nuts, raisins, coconuts, and fruits in the belief that doing so will lead to a healthy, beautiful baby.** After delivery, dried ginger powder, celery seeds, nuts, and puffed lotus seeds may be given to a new Hindu mother in an effort to cleanse her system and restore her strength. (For more on Hinduism, refer to the Religions section, later in this guide.)

▸ **Moaning and screaming are acceptable during childbirth.**

▸ **Traditionally, female relatives serve as labor partners,** though it is becoming more common for the husband to assist.

▸ **South Asian women may practice a postpartum lying-in period.** Although they are expected to feed the baby, everything else is done for them. Traditionally, female relatives take over. If none are around, the patient may expect nurses to do this.

▸ **Baby naming may be delayed for a week among Hindu Indians.** It should not be misinterpreted as a lack of bonding.

South Asian

End of Life

▸ **When a patient is diagnosed as terminal, family members may wish to shield him or her from that fact.** Upon admission (or before the need arises, if possible) ask the patient to identify how much information he or she wants regarding his or her condition, or to whom the information should be provided.

▸ **Many family members will not allow an autopsy unless it is absolutely necessary.**

Health Beliefs and Practices

▸ **Home and folk remedies are common, but their use may not be disclosed to physicians.** Explain in a nonjudgmental way that most patients try home remedies first and why it is important that you know what self-treatment regimens they have tried.

▸ **Sikhs are required not to cut their hair or shave their beards. Their hair will usually be worn in a turban. Consider this before cutting or shaving any hair in preparation for surgery.**

▸ **Observant Hindus will generally not eat meat or fish; some may not eat eggs.** Observant Muslims will not eat pork. Be sure to discuss any dietary restrictions and make sure that the dietary department is aware of them.

▸ **Muslims may not take medications, eat, or drink from sunrise to sunset during the month of Ramadan.** This period of fasting, self-sacrifice, and introspection is based on the Islamic calendar and thus occurs at a different time each year. Although they may be exempt during illness or pregnancy, they may have to make up for it later, when friends and family are not observing the practice, making it more difficult for them. Make sure the physician adjusts their medications to any changes in eating patterns.

▸ **Those who practice Ayurvedic medicine (Hindus, Sikhs, and some Muslims) classify food in terms of either hot or cold,** based on qualities inherent in the food rather than on its temperature. "Hot" foods, including meat, fish, eggs, yogurt, honey, and nuts, are encouraged for "cold" conditions, such as fever, or in anticipation of surgery, particularly in winter. "Cold" foods, such as milk, butter, cheese, fruits, and vegetables, are encouraged during the summer and for "hot" conditions, including pregnancy. Be sure to inquire about food

South Asian

preferences. (For more on Hinduism, Islam/Muslim, and Sikhism, refer to the relevant tabs in the Religions section of this guide.)

Note: Some material adapted from Zachariah R. East Indians. In Lipson JG, Dibble SL, editors: Culture & Clinical Care. *San Francisco: UCSF Nursing Press, 2005, 146–162; Rajwan RJ. South Asians. In Lipson JG, Dibble SL, Minarik PA, editors:* Culture & Clinical Care: A Pocket Guide. *San Francisco: UCSF Nursing Press, 1996, 264–279; and Hashwani SS. Pakistanis. In Lipson JG, Dibble SL, editors:* Culture & Clinical Care. *San Francisco: UCSF Nursing Press, 2005, 360–374.*

Southeast Asian

Caution: These are broad generalizations and should not be used to stereotype any individuals. They are most applicable to the least acculturated members. People from Cambodia, Laos, and Vietnam are included in this group.

Values, Worldview, and Communication

▸ **Many Southeast Asians are Buddhist** and believe in reincarnation. Many traditionalists are animists, believing that spirits inhabit objects and places and that ancestors must be worshipped so their spirits do not harm their descendants. It is not unusual for members of this cultural group to practice Christianity, however. (For more information, refer to the Buddhism tab in the Religions section of this guide.)

▸ **Modesty is highly valued,** and this value may interfere with some screening procedures, such as Pap smears and colonoscopies. Clinicians may need to take extra time to explain procedures and to accommodate modesty concerns as best as possible.

▸ **Giggling at "inappropriate" times usually indicates nervousness or discomfort.** Do not assume a lack of seriousness.

▸ **Realize that it may be difficult to obtain an accurate health history,** as patients were rarely told the name of illnesses, medicines given, or procedures performed.

Time Orientation

▸ **Present time orientation is common,** though emphasis on remembering ancestors reflects a past time orientation as well.

▸ **Older, less acculturated members may not be oriented to clock time** and may thus arrive early or late for appointments. If a specific time is important, take the time to explain that it is, and why.

Pain

▸ **This group is generally stoic.** Pay attention to nonverbal indications, such as a clenched jaw.

Family/Gender Issues

▸ **Great respect for elders is common.** Adult children are expected to care for their parents, which may interfere with their parents' self-care. If some aspects of self-care are medically necessary, give the adult children another task—such as rubbing lotion on their hands or feet—to help their parents.

Southeast Asian

- **Among older generations, men are the decision makers,** and either the husband or eldest son (if his father is deceased) may take on the role. Note that the family spokesperson may not be the decision maker, but merely the one who speaks English.
- **When a patient is accompanied by relatives,** address the eldest person present—particularly if male.

Pregnancy and Birth

- **Either the mother or her husband may be the preferred labor partner.**
- **When asked, they may not give an accurate count of pregnancies because many count only live births.**
- **Some Hmong new mothers may want to take home the placenta for burial.** If possible, honor such requests.

Pediatric

- **A baby may not be seen as "human" until several days old**—a tradition that may have developed to discourage mothers from bonding too closely in an environment with high infant mortality rates.
- **The head is the seat of life and is thus considered very personal, vulnerable, honorable, and untouchable** (except by close intimates), so avoid touching or putting intravenous lines in an infant's scalp unless necessary, and then only with explanation.
- **Some Vietnamese mothers may appear to have difficulty bonding; this is an illusion.** If they pay little attention to their newborns, it may be out of fear that if they call attention to how attractive their infant is, spirits may want to steal the child, which could result in the child's death.
- **Children may wear "spirit-strings" around their wrists or "neck rings."** Neither should be cut or removed, as some consider these to carry the children's life-souls.

Southeast Asian

End of Life

▸ **When a patient is diagnosed as terminal, family members may wish to shield him or her from that fact.** Upon admission (or before the need arises, if possible) ask patients to identify how much information they want regarding their condition, or to whom the information should be provided. Be aware that in most parts of Southeast Asia, diagnoses are usually given to the family, who decides whether to tell the patient.

▸ **Some may believe that at death parents and grandparents become ancestors,** who should be worshipped and obeyed. Because these ancestors shape the well-being of living descendants, a child (regardless of age) may have trouble agreeing to terminate the care of a parent.

▸ **Family may want to wash the body at death,** and some may want to place a coin in the deceased's mouth, according to custom.

▸ **Hmong may refuse autopsies and organ donations** because they believe that whatever is removed from the body will be missing when they are reincarnated. Ask them about their concerns.

Health Beliefs and Practices

▸ **Patients (particularly rural non-Christians) may fear surgery because many believe that souls are attached to different parts of the body. They may feel that a surgical procedure might sever this connection, thus causing illness or death.** Some may believe that if the body is cut or disfigured or parts are amputated, the patient will remain in a state of imbalance for life. This may be thought to trigger frequent illnesses for a lifetime and render the person physically incomplete in his or her next incarnation. Be sure to discuss their concerns, but don't expect to change their beliefs.

▸ **Some Hmong believe that when people are unconscious, their souls can wander, so anesthesia is dangerous.** Be sure to discuss their concerns, but don't expect to change their beliefs.

▸ **Some believe that verbal statements in and of themselves can cause illness or death** and for this reason may not want to discuss potential risks and dangers. Talk with them about their concerns.

Southeast Asian

- **Less acculturated patients may want to consult a shaman** (a traditional healer believed to have the ability to communicate with the spirit world). Allowing such consultations will generally ease their minds and increase their trust in you.
- **Therapies such as cupping and coining (or coin rubbing) are traditional remedies.** Ascertain how and why any observed markings on a patient's body were made before reporting them.
- **Some patients may have concerns about blood being drawn.** They may fear it will sap their strength, cause illness, force their souls to leave their bodies, or that it will not be replenished. If a patient is anxious, ask about his or her concerns so that they can be addressed.

Note: Information for this profile adapted from several sources, including Kulig JC, Prak S. Cambodians (Khmer). In Lipson JG, Dibble SL, editors: Culture & Clinical Care. San Francisco: UCSF Nursing Press, 2005, 73–84; Johnson SK, Hang AL. Hmong. In Lipson JG, Dibble SL, editors: Culture & Clinical Care. San Francisco: UCSF Nursing Press, 2005, 250–263; and Muecke MA. Caring for Southeast Asian refugee patients in the USA. Am J Public Health. 1983 Apr;73(4):431–438. Additional information on Hmong beliefs was taken from Fadiman A. The Spirit Catches You and You Fall Down: A Hmong Child, Her American Doctors, and the Clash of Two Cultures. New York: Farrar, Straus and Giroux, 1997.

Religions

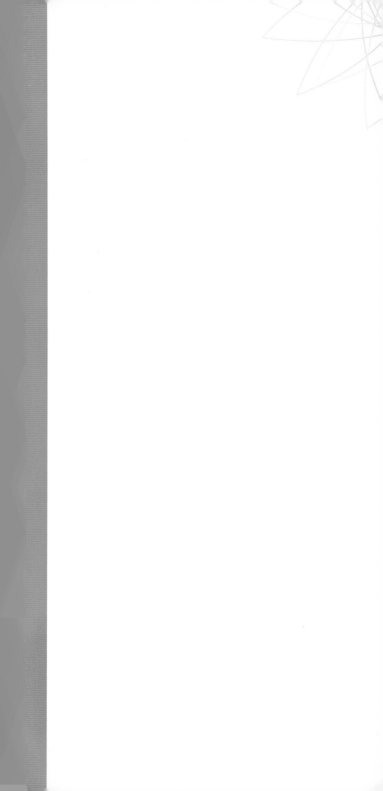

Amish

The Amish are descendants of the Christians of the "Radical Reformation" in sixteenth-century Europe. They are often confused with Mennonites, another Anabaptist (against infant baptism) group that came to the United States at the same time and are also called "Plain People." (In general, the Mennonites tend to be less restrictive and drive cars, for example, although there are some very conservative Mennonite groups and some more liberal Amish groups.) They are known for their separation from general society, their rejection of most modern technology, and their very conservative dress. Most live in Pennsylvania and in rural areas of the Midwest.

Most do not have health insurance, including Medicare, because they don't pay into Social Security. They are exempt from the Affordable Care Act. The community takes care of each other and the church will pay for any necessary medical care.

Diet

▸ There are no dietary restrictions, other than personal preference.

Healing Beliefs and Practices

▸ They usually will not seek medical care unless their ability to work is affected and the problem is quite serious.

▸ They practice faith healing and use herbal treatments. They will often seek out herbalists, reflexologists, and chiropractors before medical doctors. They believe that medicine helps, but God heals. Some may want immunizations; others won't.

▸ In general, they don't seek preventive care, both because of their faith in God and the cost of such things as immunizations, cancer screenings, Pap smears, and mammograms. They don't believe in birth control.

Medications

▸ Medications are allowed, but practitioners should be mindful that patients may not be able to keep them consistently cold (if required) due to lack of consistent electricity.

Amish

Spiritual Practices

▸ They live a very simple life and believe that their religion should be practiced, not displayed. Thus, they have little in the way of tangible religious symbols or complicated religious rituals.

▸ Young people make the decision whether to join the church or not in their late teens and early 20s. If they join, they are baptized and commit themselves to the church for the rest of their lives.

Abortion

▸ Abortion is allowed only if the mother's life is at stake.

End of Life

▸ They believe in God's will and therefore do not usually choose heroic measures, such as resuscitation. They also tend to ration care at the end of life because they don't want to waste the money of the family, the church, or the community.

▸ They prefer to die at home, cared for by the community, rather than in a hospital. Home hospice care is allowed.

Care of the Deceased

▸ The body is generally taken to a funeral home for embalming (if required by the state), and then returned to the home for a viewing so that family and members of the community may pay their respects. The body will be washed and dressed in plain clothes.

Organ Donation

▸ They are generally opposed to heart transplants, because that's where the soul resides. Other than that, organ transplants are allowed.

Autopsy

▸ Many will refuse an autopsy.

Disposition of the Body

▸ Burial usually occurs within three days of death in modest pine caskets made by the community.

Note: Much information adapted from Cleveland Clinic. Treating the Amish and Addressing Their Health Care Concerns: A Practical Guide for Health Care Providers.Oct 7, 2009. Accessed May 14, 2018. http://www.clevelandclinic.org/health/health-info/docs/1700/1783.asp?index=6955&src=newsp.

Bahá'í

The Bahá'í faith came into being in the nineteenth century and has become widespread worldwide. The central message of the religion is one of globalization and oneness of humanity. There is no clergy, only elected community spiritual assemblies.

Diet

▸ Alcohol and recreational drugs are forbidden. Otherwise, there are no dietary restrictions other than during the Nineteen Day Fast, March 2–21, which ends with the Bahá'í New Year on March 21. During that time, those between 15 and 70 years old do not drink or eat between dawn and sunset, except in the case of pregnancy, travel, or ill health.

Healing Beliefs and Practices

▸ There is harmony between science and religion, so religion should not typically pose any conflicts within health care settings. Prayer is seen to aid in healing, in addition to medical care.

Medications

▸ Narcotics are acceptable when prescribed by a physician.

Spiritual Practices

▸ Bahá'ís may want to have symbols such as the 9-pointed star; a photograph of Abdu'l-Bahá, the son of the founder/prophet; or other books of Bahá'í writings in their hospital room.

Abortion

▸ Because the soul is believed to be present from the moment of conception, abortion is strongly discouraged, but may be allowed for medical reasons.

End of Life

▸ If life support merely prolongs life in disabling illness, the decision to withhold or remove it is left to those responsible—the patient/surrogate and the physician.

Bahá'í

Care of the Deceased
- There are no formal last rites; however, family, friends, or hospital clergy may offer prayers.
- Because they believe that the soul is present from conception, an embryo/fetus should be treated with respect, and burial should be left to the discretion of the parents if possible.

Organ Donation
- Organ donation is acceptable.

Autopsy
- Autopsies are acceptable if necessary for medical or legal reasons.

Disposition of the Body
- Embalming is discouraged; cremation is strongly forbidden. Burial is preferred.

Note: Much information adapted from Metropolitan Chicago Health-care Council. Bahá'í: Guidelines for Health Care Providers Interacting with Patients of the Bahá'í Religion and Their Families. 2002. Accessed May 14, 2018. https://www.advocatehealth.com/assets/documents/faith/cgbahai.pdf.

Buddhism

Caution: These are broad generalizations and should not be used to stereotype any individuals.

Buddhism is divided into three major branches, each with its own beliefs, practices, and traditions. Each branch has numerous sub-branches and groups.

- Theravada Buddhism is practiced in Sri Lanka, Myanmar, Thailand, Laos, Cambodia, and Vietnam.
- Mahayana Buddhism is practiced in China, Korea, and Japan.
- Vajrayana Buddhism is practiced in Tibet and Japan.

With no central authority, there is a tremendous diversity in belief and practice among Buddhists. Among the common teachings is that the nature of life involves suffering, which is caused by ignorant grasping desires.

Diet
- Many Buddhists are vegetarians, but not all are. Buddhists from different branches follow different dietary rules. Be sure to discuss dietary restrictions with your patient.
- According to Buddhist teachings, the quality of your heart is more important than your diet.

Healing Beliefs and Practices
- Illness is sometimes seen as an imbalance of energy. They may perform rituals to promote healing, and some may use herbal remedies. But there are no restrictions affecting medical care.
- Artificial insemination and birth control are acceptable.
- There are no restrictions on blood or blood products.

Medications
- Some abstain from "intoxicants" that could cloud the mind, including pain medication. Some may object to medications made with animal byproducts. Check with the patient for such concerns.

Spiritual Practices
- Daily chanting of the sutras (texts of the Buddha's teaching) and other texts or meditation are common.
- Ritual objects include a set of beads on a string, used to count repeated short recitations.

Buddhism

- Soto Zen Buddhist patients (from Japan) may request a simple altar with the image of the Buddha, along with incense, a candle, and cut flowers. If candles and incense are a safety issue, fruit, sweets, and electric lights may be substituted.
- No day of the week is set aside as a special time for religious practice.

Abortion

- There is no official position on abortion. Many Buddhists believe that life begins at conception and killing is morally wrong, however, abortion is common in Japan.

Organ Donation

- It is generally acceptable to donate or receive an organ, although in some sects, individuals may be concerned that organ donation can affect the consciousness of the person who died. They would not be open to the practice.

Autopsy

- Whether autopsies are allowed is a matter of individual practice. Some Buddhists believe that consciousness remains in the body for up to three days after the patient stops breathing, so an autopsy would not be appropriate within that time frame. Check with the patient's family.

Disposition of the Body

- The family may choose burial or cremation. Cremation is common. They believe in reincarnation, so the fate of the body is less important.

End of Life

- Personal choice in the time and manner of death is of extreme importance. Death should be faced with a clear mind, even if it means experiencing pain. However, they may believe that steps should be taken to relieve pain up to this point.

Note: Much information adapted from Metropolitan Chicago Healthcare Council. Guidelines for Health Care Providers Interacting with Patients of the Buddhist Religion and Their Families. Apr 29, 2003. Accessed May 14, 2018. https://www.advocatehealth.com/assets/documents/faith/cgbuddhist.pdf.

Christian Science

Caution: These are broad generalizations and should not be used to stereotype any individuals.

The Christian Science church was established in 1879 by Mary Baker Eddy. It follows both Eddy's 1875 book, *Science and Health* and the Bible. There are no ordained clergy; elected Readers conduct services. It is based on the belief that God's creations are spiritual, rather than material. Given their beliefs regarding the nature of healing, they are less likely to seek out physicians for health care.

Diet
▸ Alcohol and tobacco are forbidden.

Healing Beliefs and Practices
▸ They believe that humans are spiritual, not physical, and therefore illness, injuries, and suffering are not "real" and can be overcome through faith and prayer. They will use dentists, optometrists, and obstetricians and will accept physical healing for something "mechanical" like a broken arm or intestinal blockage, but most healing is sought from Christian Science practitioners through prayer and counsel to remove the sick person's belief in suffering.

Medications
▸ They generally do not take medication because the path to healing is through proper mental processes.

Spiritual Practices
▸ Spiritual healing is a central focus of the religion.

Abortion
▸ The church does not tell members what position to take.

End of Life
▸ They are unlikely to seek medical help to prolong life.

Organ Donation
▸ The decision is left to the individual.

Autopsy
▸ They do not specifically object to autopsies, but they encourage participating in Western practices under special circumstances in accordance with the wishes of the deceased.

Disposition of the Body
▸ It is up to the individual.

Middle Eastern

Values, Worldview, and Communication

▸ **Effective communication is often assumed to be two-way.** You may need to share information about yourself before these patients will share information about themselves. Health care providers may be expected to take a personal interest in their patients.

▸ **Female patients may avoid direct eye contact** with health care providers of the opposite sex to avoid any hint of sexual impropriety.

▸ **Islam plays a dominant role in the lives of many Middle Easterners.** Give patients the opportunity to pray privately several times a day (five times daily is prescribed), facing east toward Mecca. Many have a fatalistic attitude regarding health (it is all in Allah's hands), so they may see their health-related behavior as being of little consequence. Inshallah means "God willing" and often follows something they hope will happen. For example, "She will recover soon, inshallah."

▸ **Repetition of demands** is often made to show emphasis, as is a loud tone of voice; it's not an attempt to annoy you.

▸ **For many Iranians, "thumbs up" is a rude gesture;** avoid using it.

Time Orientation

▸ **Arabs tend to have a past and present time orientation.** Human interaction is given higher priority than clock time; if being on time is important, emphasize it.

▸ **Iranians tend to be more future oriented,** although a fatalistic attitude can interfere with adherence to preventive medicine. Social time can be flexible.

Pain

▸ **Patients tend to be very expressive about pain,** particularly in front of family. Pain is feared and should be minimized. Explaining the source of pain and the prognosis may improve these patients' ability to cope with it.

Middle Eastern

Family/Gender Issues

▶ **Middle Easterners are very family oriented.** The family is seen as more important than the individual. Expect many familial visitors to see the patient.

▶ **Be patient with "demanding" family members.** They may see it as their job to make sure that the patient gets the best care possible.

▶ **Personal problems are usually taken care of within the family.** They may not be receptive to counseling.

▶ **Traditionally, the eldest male is the decision maker.** Even among the more acculturated, the entire family (including extended family) may participate in decision making. It may be helpful to ask in advance if there is anyone who will be making decisions with the patient who should be included in discussions.

▶ **Sexual segregation can be extremely important.** Assign same-sex caregivers whenever possible and respect a woman's modesty at all times. Offer a gown that provides maximum coverage if possible.

▶ **Accept the fact that women may defer to husbands for decision making about their own and their children's health.** In fact, the husband may answer questions addressed to his wife. This does not necessarily indicate an abusive situation.

▶ **Middle Eastern cultures are patriarchal,** and men receive more respect and status than women. Thus, male physicians may be accorded more respect.

Pregnancy and Birth

▶ **Arab women may delay prenatal care** because pregnancy is seen as a normal condition.

▶ **There may not be any plan for birth** because planning can be seen as challenging the will of Allah.

▶ **Women in labor tend to be vocally expressive of pain.** Iranian women often receive a gift of expensive jewelry to compensate for their "suffering."

▶ **A female relative may be the birth attendant;** Arab men are not expected to participate. However, acculturated Iranian men are more likely to participate.

▶ **The initial secretion from mammary glands, colostrum, is often believed to be harmful to the baby,** so breastfeeding is often delayed for the first few days. Be sure to explain the importance of colostrum to the baby's health.

Eastern Orthodox

The Eastern Orthodox Church is rooted in the New Testament Church, which was begun by Christ's disciples in accordance with his teachings. The term *Eastern* stems from the split in 1054, when the Patriarch of Rome (the center of the western portion of Constantine's empire) excommunicated the Patriarch of Constantinople (the center of the eastern portion of the empire). The Roman Catholic Church now represents the western church.

The Eastern Orthodox Church is generally known by its geographical centers, including the Greek Orthodox and Russian Orthodox Churches. They believe in the Holy Trinity—Father, Son, and Holy Spirit—three divine persons in one God, distinct but not separate.

Diet
▸ There are no dietary restrictions.
▸ Fasting from certain foods is used to strengthen the soul over the passions of the body and to encourage prayer. Such fasting may also occur at certain times of the year and before Easter for the pious.

Healing Beliefs and Practices
▸ All healing is thought to come from God; medical practitioners are seen as administrators of God's healing.
▸ Prayer, participation in the community, and the Sacraments are seen as treatments for illness.
▸ The body is seen as the temple of the Holy Spirit, and thus healing the body and the soul are directly connected.
▸ Illness of the body and human suffering are believed to have redemptive purposes.
▸ Holy Unction (anointing with oil) is administered to the sick by Orthodox clergy.

Medications and Other Medical Treatments
▸ As long as treatments do not cause harm to others, there are few restrictions.
▸ Fertility interventions that include the destruction of fertilized eggs or surrogate pregnancies are to be avoided.
▸ Animal organs should not be implanted, and fetal-cell research is forbidden.

Eastern Orthodox

Spiritual Practices
▶ Sacraments include Baptism, Repentance (Confession and Forgiveness), Communion, and Holy Unction (prayers for the sick).
▶ They attend Divine Liturgy on Sundays and/or holy days.
▶ They may pray with icons and/or incense.

Abortion
▶ Abortion is considered murder, and thus is not allowed.

End of Life
▶ Removal of "artificial" nutrition or hydration is not acceptable.
▶ Alleviation of pain is allowed only if it will in no way lead to the patient's death.
▶ A priest should be called when the patient is approaching death in order to administer Holy Communion and hear the final confession.

Care of the Deceased
▶ A priest should be notified when someone dies in order to lead those present in prayers for the release of the soul.
▶ They pray for the souls of the deceased for 40 days.

Organ Donation
▶ There are differing views on the subject of organ donation.

Autopsy
▶ Autopsies are discouraged, but not forbidden.

Disposition of the Body
▶ Embalming is discouraged, but not forbidden.
▶ Cremation is forbidden.

Hinduism

Hinduism is a religion and philosophy believed to have originated 5,000 years ago and is mainly practiced in the Indian subcontinent, Southeast Asia, Fiji, Bali, and other islands. Hindus believe in a cycle of rebirth, and each rebirth is influenced by karma (the sum of one's actions in past lives). The body is seen as a vehicle for the soul to experience the universe on its journey to God.

Diet

▶ Many are vegetarian. Some may avoid all beef products, including gelatin. Consult with the individual.
▶ If there are no dietary restrictions, some patients may want to bring food from home.
▶ Some may practice fasting on certain days, although they are generally excused from fasting if ill.

Healing Beliefs and Practices

▶ They may use alternative approaches, including Ayurvedic medicine and homeopathy. (*See also* South Asian Health Beliefs and Practices in the Cultures section of this guide.)

Medications

▶ Many may be reluctant to use medications, believing that Western medicine tends to overmedicate.
▶ Make sure the medications do not contain animal products. Those that do include heparin (anticoagulant), hepatitis A vaccine, Prevnar (pneumococcal vaccine), glucosamine (for arthritis), and many others.

Spiritual Practices

▶ They generally do not expect a visit from Hindu clergy.
▶ If possible, have copies of the *Bhagavad Gita* and other Hindu scriptures available.
▶ Some may wear a thread around their wrist or body, which has religious significance and should not be removed if possible, and not without discussion.

Abortion

▶ Except when medically indicated, it is not advised.

End of Life

▶ They tend to be accepting of natural death and are not in favor of artificially prolonging life.

Hinduism

Care of the Deceased
▸ If possible, funeral and burial arrangements should be made in advance in consultation with the family.

Organ Donation
▸ Organ donation is allowed.

Autopsy
▸ Attitudes vary. For some it is acceptable, but for others it is seen as disrespectful and disturbing to the transitioning soul.

Disposition of Body
▸ They practice cremation, preferably within 24 hours after death. The death certificate should be filled out quickly so that funeral arrangements may be completed.

Note: Much information adapted from Metropolitan Chicago Healthcare Council. Guidelines for Health Care Providers Interacting with Patients of the Hindu Religion and Their Families. Jul 10, 2002. Accessed May 14, 2018. https://www.advocatehealth.com/assets/documents/faith/cghindu.pdf.

Islam/Muslim

Caution: These are broad generalizations and should not be used to stereotype any individuals.

Muslims believe in the oneness of God and Muhammad as the last prophet of God. *Islam* means "submission" (to the will of God, or, as some interpret the word, "peace"). It is the second largest religious tradition in the world after Christianity. Although most people think of the Middle East in terms of Islam, nearly two thirds of Muslims live in the Asia-Pacific region, including Indonesia and India. Most Muslims are either Sunni (75%-90%) or Shia (10%-20%).

Diet
▸ Pork and alcohol are prohibited.
▸ Food should be halal (permissible according to Islamic law), which also takes into account the method of slaughter.
▸ During the month of Ramadan (which varies from year to year), Muslims will fast during daylight hours. Although it may be postponed during illness, many may want to fast anyway, and medications may need to be adjusted.

Healing Beliefs and Practices
▸ Prayers and reading from the Koran are used for healing. Some may carry words from the Koran.
▸ Depending on the area they're from, they may follow the cultural practice of using the right hand for eating and the left hand for toileting and hygiene.
▸ Some Muslim women may want to be examined only by female providers and may insist on covering their bodies at all times. If possible, provide modest gowns or let them wear their own, and use same-sex providers.

Medications
▸ There are no restrictions, although there may be some concern around those made with animal products. This includes heparin (anticoagulant), hepatitis A vaccine, Prevnar (pneumococcal vaccine), glucosamine (for arthritis), and many others.

Spiritual Practices
▸ The month of Ramadan (which varies each year) is a time for reflection. Muslims are required to fast from sunrise to sunset.
▸ Friday is the holy day.

Islam/Muslim

- Muslims are supposed to pray five times a day while facing Mecca (east). If possible, make sure their bed faces east. This may prevent them from getting on the floor to pray.
- They may use prayer beads to help count recitations.
- Boys are usually circumcised.

Abortion
- Abortion is forbidden after 4 months, when the fetus is thought to become a living soul. Prior to that, it is allowed only when the mother's life is in danger or in cases of rape.

End of Life
- Any attempts to shorten life are prohibited.

Care of the Deceased
- Maintaining a terminal patient on artificial life support for a prolonged period in a vegetative state is not encouraged.

Organ Donation
- Organ donation is generally acceptable.

Autopsy
- Autopsies are permitted for medical and legal purposes, otherwise forbidden, in part because it would delay burial.

Disposition of the Body
- Cremation is forbidden. The body must be washed by a same-sex Muslim at death. Burial is usually within 24 hours.

Note: Much information adapted from Metropolitan Chicago Healthcare Council. Guidelines for Health Care Providers Interacting with Muslim Patients and Their Families. Dec 8, 1999. Accessed May 14, 2018. http://gatewayeol.com/wp-content/uploads/2017/07/Islam-Guidelines-for-Health-Care-Providers-Interacting-with-Muslim-Patients-and-their-Families.pdf.

Jehovah's Witness

Caution: These are broad generalizations and should not be used to stereotype any individuals.

The Jehovah's Witness religion was founded in 1879 by Charles Taze Russell who believed that hellfire did not exist, that God was not a Trinity, and that end times were immanent.They are active evangelists and missionaries. They see themselves as Christians, but many Christians do not see them as such.

They are known in the health care community for their adherence to the New Testament command to "abstain from blood."

Diet
▸ Tobacco is forbidden; moderate alcohol is allowed.
▸ They do not eat meat from animals unless the blood has been properly drained.

Healing Beliefs and Practices
▸ They accept medical and surgical treatment, other than blood transfusions. The use of derivatives of primary blood components is left up to individual choice. Nonblood expanders are acceptable, and there are numerous alternatives to blood transfusions that may be requested. Preoperative autologous blood donations are not acceptable. Faith healing is forbidden.

Medications
▸ Medications are accepted unless they are derived from blood products. Narcotics may be given for severe pain and under the supervision of a physician; it is a personal choice.

Spiritual Practices
▸ The Sabbath is Sunday.
▸ They do not vote or serve in the military, do not celebrate traditional Christian holidays or birthdays, and do not use the symbol of the cross.
▸ Reading scriptures can comfort the individual and may lead to mental and spiritual healing. Members of the congregation and elders may visit to pray with the patient and read scriptures.

Abortion
▸ They believe that life begins at conception and are opposed to abortion.

Jehovah's Witness

End of Life
▸ They believe that life is sacred, and that reasonable efforts should be made to sustain it. However, they do not believe in taking extraordinary measures if the physician believes it would merely prolong the dying process and/or leave the patient with no quality of life.

Care of the Deceased
▸ There are no special rituals for the deceased.

Organ Donation
▸ Organ donation is seen as an individual decision; however, all blood must be removed beforehand.

Autopsy
▸ An autopsy is acceptable if required by law; however, they generally prefer to avoid it.

Disposition of the Body
▸ Either burial or cremation is acceptable.

Judaism

Caution: These are broad generalizations and should not be used to stereotype any individuals.

The Jewish religion has three designations, based on the degree of adherence to the laws of the Torah (the first five books of the Old Testament).
- Orthodox Jews (covered here) are the most adherent.
- Conservative Jews are somewhat adherent.
- Reform Jews are the least adherent.

Culturally, Sephardic Jews are those whose ancestors were expelled from Spain in 1492 and largely settled around the Mediterranean. Ashkenazi Jews are those whose ancestors are from Eastern Europe and Russia. Sephardic and Ashkenazi foods, languages, and customs differ.

The Jewish calendar is a lunisolar calendar; it is based on the phases of the moon, but a lunar month is added every two to three years to keep up with the solar calendar.

Diet
▸ Kosher laws for Orthodox and some Conservative Jews forbid pork, shellfish, and mixing of meat and dairy products. Separate (or disposable) dishes and utensils must be used for meat and dairy.

Healing Beliefs and Practices
▸ Under halacha (religious law) it is the duty of followers to do what they can to preserve and protect their lives. The saving of a life supersedes all other laws.
▸ There may be prayers for the sick. Visiting the sick is seen as a good deed (a mitzvah).
▸ Boys are circumcised on the eighth day of life.

Medications
▸ There may be concerns around medication being kosher (medications with porcine components). Although insulin is no longer made with porcine products some patients may still have that concern. Others might be concerned with the use of gelatin tablets.

Judaism

Spiritual Practices
- Yom Kippur (the date for which varies from year to year) is the Day of Atonement during which Jews are to fast and do no work from sunset to the following sundown.
- The Sabbath is sundown Friday to one hour past sundown Saturday. Orthodox Jews will avoid all "work," including ringing the call button, signing forms, or exchanging money.
- Orthodox men may wear a prayer shawl, *yarmulke* (skull cap), and tefillin (black leather boxes with straps that Orthodox Jewish men wear during weekday morning prayer).
- Jews believe each individual relates directly to God; no intermediary is necessary for prayer.

Abortion
- Abortion is sanctioned as a means of safeguarding the life and well-being of the mother.
- Reform and Conservative movements advocate a woman's right to safe and accessible abortions.

End of Life
- There is an obligation to preserve and protect life.
- Withdrawing a "cyclical" treatment such as chemotherapy may be permitted, whereas withdrawing life support (a "continuous" treatment) is generally problematic.

Care of the Deseased
- When someone dies, the body is to be washed and dressed by someone Jewish in accordance with prescribed ritual. If hospital staff must touch the body, they should wear gloves. Someone should sit with the body after death.

Organ Donation
- Organ donation is a complicated issue, based on, among other things, the interpretation of the principle that the body of the dead may not be used for the benefit of the living and concern with tampering with a corpse unless it is to directly save a life. Will all organs be used for immediate transplant?
- Many Jewish authorities maintain that if the heart is still beating, the patient is alive, even if brain-dead. Thus, to remove an organ while the heart is still beating is tantamount to murder. However, most Reform and Conservative movements support it, and the Orthodox community is coming to accept it.

Judaism

Autopsy

▶ Autopsies are somewhat problematic; however, they are permitted if required by law.

Disposition of the Body

▶ Bodies should be buried, not cremated. Cremation is seen as inappropriate. Burial should take place within 24 hours.

▶ All body parts, including bloody clothing and amputated limbs, should be buried with body.

Note: Much information adapted from Metropolitan Chicago Healthcare Council. Guidelines for Health Care Providers Interacting with Jewish Patients and Their Families. Feb 15, 2002. Accessed May 14, 2018. https://www.advocatehealth.com/assets/documents/faith/cgjewish.pdf.

Hispanic/Latino

Caution: These are broad generalizations and should not be used to stereotype any individuals. They are most applicable to the least acculturated members. Although many of the patterns described are common to many Latin and Central Americans, they are most applicable to Mexicans.

Values, Worldview, and Communication

▸ **Personal relationships are valued.** Asking about the patient's family and interests before focusing on health issues will generally increase rapport and trust.

▸ **Patients may have a fatalistic view of the world,** which can interfere with preventive behavior. It may be necessary to spend extra time explaining why preventive behavior is important.

Time Orientation

▸ **Many people in this culture have a present time orientation, which may impede preventive medicine and follow-up care.** Explain the need for preventive medication (such as for hypertension) and to finish antibiotics even after symptoms have disappeared. Using analogies can be helpful. Tie adherence to something the patient cares about (for example, dancing at a daughter's wedding or holding a grandchild).

Pain

▸ **While patients may tend to be expressive (loud) when in pain,** males may be more expressive around family members than around health care professionals. Do not make the mistake of stereotyping Hispanic patients as "loud" and thus ignore a real medical problem.

Family/Gender Issues

▸ **Large numbers of family members may visit the patient.** It is a cultural way to express love and concern. Allow family members to spend as much time as possible with the patient. Allow them to assist the patient with the activities of daily living if the patient is reluctant to do self-care.

▸ **Realize that patients may not want to discuss emotional problems outside the family.**

▸ **Modesty is important,** particularly among older women; try to keep them covered whenever possible.

▸ **Accept that more traditional wives, especially recent immigrants, may defer to husbands in decision making,** both for their own health and for that of their children. When a patient comes in, find out with whom he or she may want to consult before making decisions.

Hispanic/Latino

Pregnancy and Birth

▸ **Pregnancy is seen as a normal condition,** so prenatal care may not be sought.

▸ **The woman's mother may be the preferred birthing partner.**

▸ **Laboring women may be quite vocally expressive,** while others may be surprisingly stoic.

▸ **Traditionally, new mothers avoid cold, bathing, and exercise for six weeks postpartum.** Respect postpartum prescriptions for rest. Sponge baths may be preferred.

▸ **Pregnancy is considered a "hot" condition;** birth is thought to deplete the body of heat. Restoration of warmth is important. Offer liquids other than ice water, which may be deemed too "cold."

▸ **The initial secretion from mammary glands, colostrum, may be seen as "bad" or "spoiled" milk and thus harmful to the baby,** so breastfeeding is often delayed for the first few days. Be sure to explain the importance of colostrum to the baby's health.

Pediatric

▸ **There are a number of folk diseases that affect children,** including *mal de ojo* (evil eye), *caída de la mollera* (fallen fontanelle, often caused by dehydration), and *empacho* (stomach pain).

▸ **"Evil eye" is generally believed to be caused by envy when someone compliments a child.** Be sure to touch the child when complimenting him or her to prevent this. The child may be wearing a red string or "deer's eye" (a large brown seed with red string) to prevent it.

▸ **Herbal remedies are often used.** Be sure to ask about them. Chamomile tea (*manzanilla*), used to treat colic, is generally safe and sometimes helpful. However, *greta*, a yellow to grayish-yellow powder, and *azarcón*, a bright reddish-orange powder, both of which are used to treat *empacho* (stomach pain), contain lead and can be dangerous.

▸ **A chubby baby is seen as a healthy baby,** so additional teaching regarding diet and diabetes may be warranted.

▸ **When a baby has a fever, he or she will often be bundled up,** which may run counter to cooling measures that may have been instructed. Be sure to explain the rationale for the cooling measures without disrespecting cultural beliefs.

Hispanic/Latino

- **It is important to include the grandmother in patient teaching,** because she may have the most to say in terms of day-to-day health care issues, particularly if she lives with the family.
- **Belly button binders may be used to prevent an "outie."** Your concerns should be with the cleanliness of the coin and the tightness of the binder. Instead of advising caregivers not to use a binder, teach them to make sure the coin is clean and that the binder is not too tight.

End of Life

- **When a patient is diagnosed as terminal, family members may wish to shield him or her from that fact.** Upon admission (or before the need arises, if possible), ask patients how much information they want regarding their condition, or to whom the information should be provided. Family members may resist hospice for fear it will emphasize the fact that their loved one is dying and thus encourage the individual to give up hope and lose the will to live. Be sure to ask about their concerns so you can address them.
- **The family of a terminal patient may be reluctant to remove life support lest it be seen as encouraging death.** If the illness is determined to be "punishment by God," life support may be considered interfering with the opportunity for the patient to redeem his or her sins through suffering. At the same time, however, traditional respect and courtesy toward physicians may lead the patient or the patient's family to agree with a physician who suggests removing life support, even when they are opposed to it. It may be helpful to say, "I know that some people have serious concerns about removing life support. Do you share those concerns? May we talk about them?"

Health Beliefs and Practices

- **A predominant theory of illness is that it results from an upset in body balance.** Patients may refuse certain foods or medications that upset the hot/cold body balance, even if they do not verbalize it as such. With this in mind, offer alternative foods and liquids. Ask if they prefer water with ice or at room temperature.
- **Among those following traditional cultural practices, fat is seen as healthy.** Many Mexican foods are high in fat and salt. Because of this, nutritional counseling may be necessary for diabetics and individuals with high blood pressure or heart disease. There are

Hispanic/Latino

"heart-healthy" Mexican cookbooks and online recipes available.

▸ **Ask what remedies the patient tried before coming in.** Ask in a way that implies that all your patients attempt self-treatment before coming in and that you need to know about those attempts to avoid prescribing something that could cause a bad interaction. Do not let the patient believe you are criticizing him or her for trying home remedies or seeing other healers. Doing so might lessen the patient's trust in you.

Mormonism
The Church of Jesus Christ of
Latter-Day Saints

Caution: These are broad generalizations and should not
be used to stereotype any individuals.

The Church of Jesus Christ of Latter-Day Saints (LDS) was
founded in 1830, after the Angel Moroni appeared to
Joseph Smith and led him to the golden plates containing
the revelations of many prophets. He translated them into
English, and they became the Book of Mormon.

Utah is the center of Mormon cultural influence and are
active proselytizers. They practiced polygamy during the
nineteenth century.

They keep meticulous genealogical records for the practice of baptism of the dead (see Spiritual Practices below).

Diet
▸ Alcohol, tobacco, coffee, and tea are forbidden.
▸ They generally live a healthy lifestyle.

Healing Beliefs and Practices
▸ Prayer may be used for healing, even though physical
  healing may not be part of God's plan at the time.
▸ Birth control and sterilization are strongly discouraged,
  not surprisingly, given their strong orientation
  toward family.

Medications
▸ There are no restrictions on prescribed drugs,
  although illegal drugs are forbidden. They may use
  herbal remedies.

Spiritual Practices
▸ Baptism takes place after the age of 8, which is the age
  of accountability. Baptism is seen as essential to salva-
  tion, yet not everyone who has ever lived will have had
  the opportunity to hear Christ's gospel and be
  baptized, so proxy baptisms are performed on behalf of
  those who have already died, and the dead can choose
  whether or not to accept it.
▸ The Sabbath is Sunday.
▸ Adult members of the church wear special undergar-
  ments ("the garment") that is considered sacred;
  individuals may not want to remove it. Discuss it with
  them first.

Mormonism
The Church of Jesus Christ of Latter-Day Saints

Abortion

▸ When done for personal or social convenience, it warrants excommunication; however, it can be justified when pregnancy threatens the life of the mother or is the result of rape or incest.

End of Life

▸ There are no special rituals for the dying, but the local bishop can be contacted to say prayers. If death is inevitable, promote a peaceful and dignified death.

Care of the Deceased

▸ If the sacred "garment" has been worn in life, the individual should be dressed in it once the body has been prepared for transfer to the mortuary.

Organ Donation

▸ Organ donations are allowed and seen as a selfless act.

Autopsy

▸ Autopsies are permitted with the consent of the family.

Disposition of the Body

▸ **Cremation is discouraged; burial is more common. The decision is left to the family.**

Note: Much information adapted from Ashford and St. Peter's Hospitals. Caring for the Mormon Patient. Accessed May 14, 2018. https://www.ashfordstpeters.info/images/other/PAS11.pdf; and Church of Jesus Christ of Latter-Day Saints. 21.3 Medical and Health Policies. In Handbook 2: Administering the Church. Accessed May 14, 2018. https://www.lds.org/handbook/handbook-2-administering-the-church/selected-church-policies/21.3?lang=eng&_r=1#213.

Protestantism

Caution: These are broad generalizations and should not be used to stereotype any individuals.

There are several Protestant denominations in the United States, including Baptist, Episcopalian, Lutheran, Methodist, and Presbyterian. This form of Christianity began during the Reformation as a movement against perceived errors in the Roman Catholic Church.

They believe in the Trinity, but reject the papacy and believe in the priesthood of all believers, although there is disagreement in the details among the different sects. There is much variation in terms of how literally they adhere to the Bible.

Diet
▸ There are no general dietary restrictions.
▸ Some have days of fasting.

Health Beliefs and Practices
▸ Medical decisions are an individual choice.
▸ There are prayers for healing.
▸ There is much variation in terms of beliefs regarding the cause of illness. Some may see it as punishment for sin, or as a test from God. Others see it as part of the natural course of events.

Medications
▸ There are no general guidelines, although some denominations may have suggestions and restrictions.
▸ In general, they are receptive to modern medical care.

Spiritual Practices
▸ Prayer, anointing, Eucharist, or other rituals may be important.
▸ Some may have clergy or others come to the hospital to pray with the patient.
▸ Some, though not all, practice infant baptism.

Abortion
▸ Varies. Some denominations support abortion rights with limits, others with few or no limits.

End of Life
▸ Withdrawal of treatment is an individual issue.
▸ End-of-life issues vary for each person.
▸ Euthanasia decisions vary from individual decision to religious restrictions.
▸ Most are in favor of writing advance directives.

Protestantism

Care of the Deceased
▸ **Some may practice anointing with oil.**
▸ Prayers or reading of scriptures may be appreciated.

Organ Donation
▸ Typically, organ donation is an individual decision.

Autopsy
▸ The decision whether to have an autopsy or not is usually made by the family.

Disposition of the Body
▸ **Whether the body is cremated or buried is the decision of the family.**

Note: Much information adapted from Metropolitan Chicago Healthcare Council. Quick Reference for Health Care Providers Interacting with Protestant Patients and Their Families. Mar 23, 2005. Accessed May 14, 2018. http://www.marianjoylibrary.org/Diversity/ documents/qrprotestant.pdf; and Prezi Inc. Protestant Views on Healthcare. Kelley E. Sep 13, 2013. Accessed May 14, 2018. https:// prezi.com/ah77zju1t9pz/protestant-views-on-healthcare/.

Roman Catholicism

Caution: These are broad generalizations and should not be used to stereotype any individuals.

One of three major forces of Christianity (along with Protestantism and Eastern Orthodoxy), Roman Catholicism is distinguished from other forms of Christianity by its beliefs, practices, and traditions.

They believe in the special authority of the Pope, the ability of saints to intercede on behalf of believers, and the doctrine of transubstantiation (wherein the bread of the Eucharist becomes the true body of Christ when blessed by a priest). Worship tends to be more formal and ritualized. They believe in the Holy Trinity of the Father (God), the Son (Jesus Christ), and the Holy Spirit.

Diet

▸ Traditionally, Catholics have abstained from eating meat on Ash Wednesday, which varies from year to year, and on Fridays during the season of Lent. Catholics are also expected to fast on Ash Wednesday and Good Friday.

Healing Beliefs and Practices

▸ They believe in the power of God to heal. Before surgery or when ill, sacraments and a blessing by a Catholic priest are important. The sacrament historically referred to as "last rites" is now positioned by the Catholic Church as a sacrament for the sick, not necessarily for the dying. Patients may ask for the sacrament of the Anointing of the Sick, when ill.

Medications

▸ Birth control is officially forbidden, although birth control pills may be allowed when they are necessary for medical reasons (most commonly for endometriosis). Today, many Catholics do use contraceptives.

Spiritual Practices

▸ The Lord's Day is on Sunday.
▸ Religious objects include the crucifix, rosary beads (a loop of beads on a string with a crucifix, used for prayer), scapular (a small cloth devotional pendant), and religious medals. Patients may want to keep such items with them during medical procedures. Discuss the option of putting them in a sealed bag kept on or near the patient.

Abortion

▸ They are opposed to abortion in all circumstances.

Roman Catholicism

End of Life
▸ They are obligated to take ordinary, not extraordinary, means to prolong life.

Care of the Deceased
▸ No special preparation of the body is requested.

Organ Donation
▸ Organ donation is allowed. It is seen as an act of charity and love.

Autopsy
▸ Autopsies are allowed.

Disposition of the Body
▸ Burial is usually preferred, although cremation is now acceptable.

Seventh-Day Adventism

Caution: These are broad generalizations and should not be used to stereotype any individuals.

Seventh-day Adventism is an end times church founded in 1863. They generally hold the writings of Ellen G. White as the authoritative, inspired word of God although they also consider the Bible a sacred text. They see themselves as Christians, but many Christians do not see them as such.

They believe in the imminent Second Coming (advent) of Jesus Christ. They believe that the soul is mortal and after death, will "sleep" in the grave until the resurrection at Christ's second coming. At that time, the redeemed will receive eternal life.

Diet
▸ A vegetarian diet is encouraged. Alcohol, coffee, and tea are prohibited.

Healing Beliefs and Practices
▸ Family planning is seen as a responsibility, and thus contraception is allowed.
▸ Healthful living is a moral obligation. Air, sunlight, rest, exercise, proper diet, and trust in divine power are seen as true remedies.

Medications
▸ There are no restrictions on medications.

Spiritual Practices
▸ The Sabbath is from sundown Friday to sundown Saturday. Elective diagnostic services and therapies should be avoided during the Sabbath.

Abortion
▸ Abortions should be performed only for serious reasons, not for gender selection, birth control, or convenience. Such serious reasons include threat to the pregnant woman's life or health, severe congenital defects, and when pregnancy results from rape or incest. The final decision is up to the woman after appropriate consultation; she should not be coerced into any position because that would infringe on her personal freedom.

Seventh-Day Adventism

End of Life

▸ They support the use of modern medicine to extend life; however, when it becomes clear that medical treatment cannot save a patient, they believe care should shift to relieve suffering. They follow state laws in determining death.

Care of the Deceased

▸ No special rituals are conducted with the deceased. It is up to the individual family.

Organ Donation

▸ Organ donation is acceptable. Adventists owned and operated Loma Linda University in California, where infant heart transplant surgery was pioneered.

Autopsy

▸ Autopsies are allowed.

Disposition of the Body

▸ Burial and cremation are both acceptable.

Note: Much information adapted from Park Ridge Center for the Study of Health, Faith, and Ethics. The Seventh-day Adventist Tradition: Religious Beliefs and Healthcare Decisions. DuBose ER, editor; Walters JW. 2002. Accessed May 14, 2018. http://www.trinity-health.org/documents/Ethics/4%20Religious%20Traditions/Adventism/Seventh%20Day%20Adventist.pdf.

Sikhism

Caution: These are broad generalizations and should not be used to stereotype any individuals.

The Sikh faith, founded in the Punjab region of India, is the fifth largest religion in the world. They believe in one, universal, formless God who is the creator of the universe and all living things.

The word *Sikh* means "disciple." They follow a path of meditation on God's name, earning an honest living, sharing good fortune with the needy, and serving humanity selflessly.

They are usually recognized by their turbans, which, along with men's beards, lead them to be confused with Muslims.

Diet

▸ Intoxicants, including alcohol, tobacco, and illicit drugs, are forbidden. Many do not eat beef due to a ban on eating meat that has been ritually slaughtered or prepared for another religion (for example, kosher or halal meat). Some Sikhs will extend this rule to all meat and meat products, and even eggs, fish, and dairy products.
▸ When Sikhs are confused with Muslims, they may be offered halal food by well-meaning staff. This can be problematic.
▸ Vegetarian or non-vegetarian meals are an individual preference.

Healing Beliefs and Practices

▸ Sikhs will combine prayer with Western medicine, herbs, and other alternative therapies, although some may accept the will of God rather than following recommended medical treatment. They may play sacred music.
▸ Their body hair is not to be cut or shaved. If it is necessary for medical reasons, be sure to consult the patient and get permission. The patient may refuse, in which case try to make appropriate adaptions.
▸ They value cleanliness; daily bathing and personal hygiene will be appreciated.
▸ Same-sex providers are often preferred.

Medications

▸ There are no restrictions on medications.

Sikhism

Spiritual Practices
- The Sikh articles of faith include the Kesh (uncut hair), which is kept covered by a distinctive turban, the Kirpan (sword), Kara (metal bracelet), Kanga (comb), and Kachera (undershorts).
- It is a cultural and religious practice to visit the sick, so expect visitors.

Abortion
- Abortion is not advised, although it is allowed for medical indications. It is not uncommon among the Sikh community in India.

End of Life
- Death is seen as a natural process and God's will. Prayer and meditation on the scripture is extremely important.

Care of the Deceased
- The five articles of faith must remain on the body. Prayers and hymns may continue. The body will be washed in a yogurt and redressed with the five articles of faith.

Organ Donation
- Organ transplants are acceptable.

Autopsy
- Autopsies are permitted.

Disposition of the Body
- Cremation is generally preferred and should take place as soon as possible after death.

Note: Much information adapted from Metropolitan Chicago Healthcare Council. Guidelines for Health Care Providers Interacting with Patients of the Sikh Religion and Their Families. Nov 29, 2000. Accessed May 14, 2018. https://www.kyha.com/assets/docs/PreparednessDocs/cg-sikh.pdf.

Additional Resources

General

Alberta Health Services. Health Care and Religious Beliefs, 2nd ed. 2015. Accessed May 14, 2018. https://www.albertahealthservices.ca/assets/programs/ps-1026227-health-care-religious-beliefs.pdf.

Arritt T. Caring for . . . patients of different religions. Nursing Made Incredibly Easy. 2014 Nov–Dec;12(6):38–45. Accessed May 14, 2018. https://journals.lww.com/nursingmadeincrediblyeasy/Fulltext/2014/11000/Caring_for___Patients_of_different_religions.8.aspx.

Ehman, J. Religious Diversity: Practical Points for Health Care Providers, rev. ed. Hospital of the University of Pennsylvania, Department of Pastoral Care. May 8, 2012. Accessed May 14, 2018. http://www.uphs.upenn.edu/pastoral/resed/Diversity_GUIDE_for_staff_rev_2012.pdf.

Greater Manchester Mental Health. The Handbook of Faiths and Cultures. Accessed May 14, 2018. https://www.gmmh.nhs.uk/download.cfm?doc=docm93jijm4n901.pdf&ver=1686.

HealthCare Chaplaincy. A Dictionary of Patients' Spiritual & Cultural Values for Health Care Professionals. (Updated: Jul 2011.) Accessed May 14, 2018. http://www.healthcarechaplaincy.org/userimages/A%20Dictionary%20of%20Patients%27%20Spiritual%20%20Cultural%20Values%20for%20Health%20Care%20Professionals_%20July%202011.pdf.

HealthCare Chaplaincy. Handbook of Patients' Spiritual and Cultural Values for Health Care Professionals. (Updated: Mar 2013.) Accessed May 14, 2018. http://www.healthcarechaplaincy.org/userimages/Cultural%20Sensitivity%20handbook%20from%20HealthCare%20Chaplaincy%20%20%283-12%202013%29.pdf.

Loma Linda University Health System. Health Care and Religious Beliefs. Accessed May 14, 2018. https://semhca.weebly.com/uploads/1/3/4/4/13445948/healthcare-religious-beliefs.pdf.

Religion Facts. Home page. Accessed May 14, 2018 http://www.religionfacts.com

Religion Facts. List of Religions & Belief Systems. Mar 17, 2004. (Updated: Feb 1, 2017.) Accessed April 14, 2018. http://www.religionfacts.com/religions.

On Abortion

Orthodox Church in America. Orthodox Christians and Abortion. Garvey J. Jan 18, 2013. Accessed May 14, 2018. https://oca.org/the-hub/the-church-on-current-issues/orthodox-christians-and-abortion.

Pew Research Center. Religious Groups' Official Positions on Abortion. Jan 16, 2013. Accessed May 14, 2018. http://www.pewforum.org/2013/01/16/religious-groups-official-positions-on-abortion/.

Pew Research Center. Where Major Religious Groups Stand on Abortion. Masci D. Jun 21, 2016. Accessed May 14, 2018. http://www.pewresearch.org/fact-tank/2016/06/21/where-major-religious-groups-stand-on-abortion/.

On Autopsies

Medscape. Religions and the Autopsy. Burton EC. (Updated: Mar 20, 2012.) Accessed May 14, 2018. https://emedicine.medscape.com/article/1705993-overview#a3.

On Diet

Deseret News. Dietary Guidelines of Some of the World's Major Religions. Purdy A. May 23, 2012. Accessed May 14, 2018. https://www.deseretnews.com/top/714/0/Dietary-guidelines-of-some-of-the-worlds-major-religions.html.

On End-of-Life Care

The Alfred Hospital. Multicultural Care at the Time of Death and Dying: A Look at the Needs of Patients & Families in the Hospital Situation. Leeming K, Hope M. Accessed May 14, 2018. http://www.alfredicu.org.au/assets/Documents/ICU-Guidelines/DeathAndDying/CALDMulticulturalCareDeathDying.pdf.

University of Massachusetts Medical School, Lamar Soutter Library. Cultural Approaches to Pediatric Palliative Care in Central Massachusetts: Protestant. (Updated: Sep 14, 2017.) Accessed May 14, 2018. https://libraryguides.umassmed.edu/c.php?g=499760&p=3422629.

Romain M, Sprung CL. End-of-life practices in the intensive care unit: The importance of geography, religion, religious affiliation, and culture. Rambam Maimonides Med J. 2014 Jan;5(1):e0003. Accessed May 14,

2018. https://www.ncbi.nlm.nih.gov/pmc/articles/PMC3904478/.

On Funerals

Everplans. Eastern Orthodox Funeral Traditions. Accessed May 14, 2018. https://www.everplans.com/articles/eastern-orthodox-funeral-traditions.

The Funeral Source. Funeral Traditions: Religious Traditions. Accessed May 14, 2018. http://thefuneralsource.org/trad02.html.

Orthodox Church in America. Cremation. Accessed May 14, 2018. https://oca.org/questions/deathfunerals/cremation.

On Medicines/Pharmaceuticals

Queensland Department of Health. Guideline: Medicines/Pharmaceuticals of Animal Origin. Document #QH-GDL-954. Jan 11, 2013. Accessed May 14, 2018. https://www.health.qld.gov.au/__data/assets/pdf_file/0024/147507/qh-gdl-954.pdf.

St. Andrew Greek Orthodox Church. Organ Donation and Transplants. Jun 22, 2017. Accessed May 14, 2018. http://saintandrewgoc.org/home/2017/6/22/organ-donation-and-transplants.

On Organ Donation

Finger Lakes Donor Recovery Network. Religion and Organ Donation. Accessed May 14, 2018. http://www.donorrecovery.org/learn/religion-and-organ-donation/.

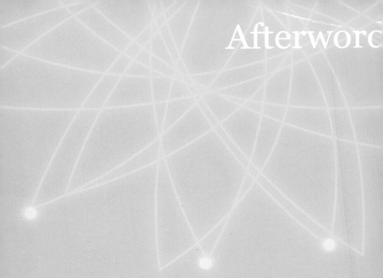

A Word from The Joint Commission

Cultural and Religious Sensitivity: A Pocket Guide for Health Care Professionals from Joint Commission Resources highlights the importance of incorporating the patient's cultural and religious perspective into his or her health care and provides helpful information to health care professionals as they strive to meet each patient's unique needs.

The Joint Commission is committed to improving communication and patient- and family-centered care.

Over the years, The Joint Commission has engaged in many activities and initiatives to better understand the issues of cultural and religious sensitivity and how they intersect with other aspects of communication and patient- and family-centered care:

▸ Comparison of Joint Commission accreditation standards to the Office of Minority Health's National Standards for Culturally and Linguistically Appropriate Services (CLAS)

▸ *Hospitals, Language, and Culture: A Snapshot of the Nation (HLC)*, a research study focused on culturally and linguistically diverse patient populations

▸ *"What Did the Doctor Say?": Improving Health Literacy to Protect Patient Safety*, a public policy white paper